bridging
responses

A front-line worker's guide
to supporting women who
have post-traumatic stress

Lori Haskell

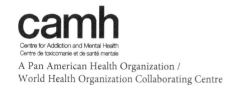

A Pan American Health Organization /
World Health Organization Collaborating Centre

Bridging responses: A front-line worker's guide to supporting women who have post-traumatic stress

ISBN: 978-1-77052-261-9 (PRINT)

Printed in Canada
Copyright © 2001 Centre for Addiction and Mental Health

No part of this work may be reproduced or transmitted in any form or by any means electronic or mechanical, including photocopying and recording, or by any information storage and retrieval system without written permission from the publisher — except for a brief quotation (not to exceed 200 words) in a review or professional work.

This book was produced by:

DEVELOPMENT
Julia Greenbaum, CAMH

EDITORIAL
Sue McCluskey, CAMH
Mark Leger

DESIGN
Eva Katz, CAMH
Nancy Leung, CAMH

PRINT PRODUCTION
Christine Harris, CAMH

MARKETING
Bernard King, CAMH

This publication may be available in other formats. For information about alternative formats or other CAMH publications, or to place an order, please contact CAMH Publications:
Toll-free: 1 800 661-1111
Toronto: 416 595-6059
E-mail: publications@camh.ca
Online store: http://store.camh.ca

Web site: www.camh.ca

2612 / 09-2016 / PG112

ACKNOWLEDGMENT

Writer:
Lori Haskell EDD C.PSYCH.

Centre for Addiction and Mental Health project team:
Barbara Dorian MD FRCPC
Julia Greenbaum MA
Ursula Kasperowski EDD C.PSYCH.
Ellie Munn BSW

Gratitude is extended to the following reviewers for providing helpful feedback on earlier versions of this booklet:

Joanne Bacon, Program Manager, Women with Disabilities and Deaf Women's Program, Education Wife Assault, Toronto, Ontario

Laurie Charlton, Elizabeth Fry Society, Toronto, Ontario

Michelle Combs, Sistering, Toronto, Ontario

Julie Dykerman, Street Haven Case Management, Toronto, Ontario

Jenny Horseman, Literacy Consultant, Toronto, Ontario

Ann Kerr, Sheena's Place, Toronto, Ontario

Adrianna LeBlanc, Community Resources Consultants of Toronto, Toronto, Ontario

Myra Lefkowitz, Community Safety Co-ordinator, University of Toronto, Toronto, Ontario

Alex Maattanen, CONTACT Mental Health Outreach Service, St Michael's Hospital, Toronto, Ontario

Treanor Mahood-Greer, Community Counselling Centre of Nipissing, North Bay, Ontario

Cathy McGrady, Mental Health Emergency Crisis Team, Sunnybrook and Women's College Health Sciences Centre, Toronto, Ontario

Cherie Miller, Jean Tweed Centre, Toronto, Ontario

Melanie Randall, Centre for Research on Violence Against Women and Children, University of Western Ontario, London, Ontario

Teresa Roberson, Sistering, Toronto, Ontario

A special thanks to staff of *Women's Health in Women's Hands*, a women's health centre in Toronto, for providing subjects and a setting for the photos used in this booklet.

contents

III Acknowledgment

OVERVIEW
1 Who is this guide for?
1 What is the guide about?
2 What is post-traumatic stress?
4 Abuse, violence and post-traumatic stress in women's lives
6 Different kinds of post-traumatic stress — simple and complex
7 Why do we need to know about complex post-traumatic stress disorder?
11 Trauma in a biopsychosocial framework

HELPFUL INTERVENTIONS FOR FRONT-LINE WORKERS
15 What can you offer as a front-line worker?
16 Recognizing the signs of post-traumatic stress responses
18 How to screen for post-traumatic stress responses
20 Actively facilitating abuse disclosures: finding the balance
22 Helpful questions for post-traumatic stress response screening
23 Be prepared for and be sensitive to clients' responses

TREATMENT APPROACHES
25 Therapeutic options
26 When medication might be helpful
26 The importance of referrals
27 Collaborative approaches
27 A hopeful concluding note

FURTHER READING
29 For understanding trauma
30 Sources for survivors
30 References

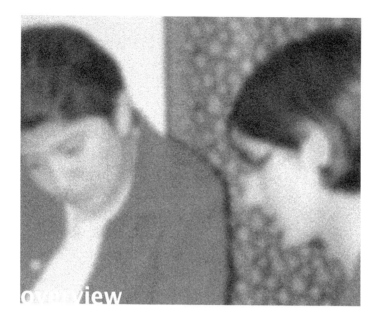

overview

WHO IS THIS GUIDE FOR?

This guide is for people working on the "front lines" — general practitioners, nurses, police officers, and those working in community health agencies, hospitals, public health services or emergency room settings, clinics and shelters that provide direct services to women. It provides general information to help you identify and understand post-traumatic stress resulting from abuse or violence. It also provides guidelines for asking about these issues so you can offer clients assistance and referral information.

WHAT IS THE GUIDE ABOUT?

There is an increased awareness in the mental health field that many women who seek treatment for depression, suicidal feelings, substance use problems, difficult or abusive relationships, and self-inflicted harm are experiencing post-traumatic stress or complex post-traumatic stress responses. Most often, these problems arise from a history of chronic child abuse or neglect.

Women experiencing post-traumatic stress may seek help from a number of services. This guide was written with a diverse audience in mind. Front-line workers may need background information that explains some of the complex responses they hear from trauma survivors. Many of the physiological, psychological and other responses of your clients may actually be the effects of trauma.

We hope this guide will serve as a quick reference to help you recognize the signs of post-traumatic stress responses.

Some front-line service providers are unsure of their role when working with women they suspect to be experiencing post-traumatic stress.

The challenge for service providers on the front lines is that their contact with trauma survivors is often brief. As a result, they understandably worry about raising such a sensitive topic with their women clients if they can't provide ongoing therapy or support.

THE PURPOSE OF THIS GUIDE IS TO HELP YOU

- Recognize the signs of post-traumatic stress from what may seem to be an array of unrelated symptoms/problems.
- Screen for and discuss, in a respectful, non-threatening and caring way, post-traumatic stress with women who may have a history of violence and abuse.
- Establish a level of safety and confidence that encourages a trauma survivor to seek help from appropriate services or resources.
- Respond appropriately, and direct trauma survivors toward further sources of help and services.
- Support the client and practise *active facilitation* by respectfully responding to the client's disclosures.

WHAT IS POST-TRAUMATIC STRESS?

Post-traumatic stress is the result of exposure to a traumatic or extremely emotionally and psychologically distressing event or events. Traumatic experiences have traditionally been defined as life-threatening.

Many women who experience post-traumatic stress, however, do not think their experiences were that serious. Furthermore, the traditional definition doesn't capture the experiences of countless women who survived not only past or present physical and sexual abuse, but also childhood neglect and emotional abuse.

A more complete definition is as follows: *a traumatic experience is an event that continues to exert negative effects on thinking (cognition), feelings (affect) and behaviour, long after the event is in the past.*

Post-traumatic stress is referred to as *post-traumatic stress disorder* (PTSD) in the clinical literature. However, labelling the symptoms of post-traumatic stress as a "disorder" may have the unintended effect of *pathologizing* (attributing problems to a "pathology" or innate disorder in) those affected by trauma.

Women who have experienced abuse, or other traumatic events, should not be stigmatized. Instead, it is important to recognize that the effects and symptoms of abuse-related trauma are themselves normal responses. They are ways of coping with the harm inflicted by the abuse.

There is valuable information in the clinical literature dealing with the treatment of PTSD. Where it is necessary for clinical accuracy, then, this guide will make use of the term PTSD. However, because language is so important and the need to avoid pathologizing women is so critical, the effects of trauma are mostly described in this guide by a new and slightly modified term — *post-traumatic stress responses* (PTSR).

People react to traumatic experiences in vastly different ways. Some of the responses are obvious, such as intrusive memories or panic attacks. Other responses, such as feeling numb and empty, are subtle and difficult to identify.

These responses may continue for years following the traumatic event or events or, in some cases, responses may subside and return later, which is often the case with survivors of childhood abuse.

While the outward display of PTSR varies widely, three categories — or "clusters" — of responses are associated with post-traumatic stress:

- reliving the event through recurring nightmares, flashbacks or other intrusive images that "pop" into one's head at any time. People who experience PTSR may also have extreme emotional or physical reactions, such as uncontrollable shaking, chills or heart palpitations, or panic when faced with reminders of the event.
- avoiding reminders of the event, inclu-ding places, people, thoughts or other activities associated with the trauma. People who experience PTSR become emotionally numb, withdraw from friends and family and lose interest in everyday activities.
- being on guard or *hyper-aroused* at all times, including irritability or sudden anger, difficulty sleeping, lack of con-centration, being overly alert or easily startled.

ABUSE, VIOLENCE AND POST-TRAUMATIC STRESS IN WOMEN'S LIVES

In recent years, we have come to realize that many women seeking help from front-line services have experienced some form of violence as children and/or as adults. The complexity of the long-term effects of this violence, though, is not often fully recognized. This includes, most importantly, PTSR.

The developmental, emotional and psychological consequences of violence and trauma are often underestimated, and often misunderstood. Yet it is imperative that those providing service to women with abuse histories be sensitive to the impact of trauma so they can steer them toward appropriate sources of help.

DIFFERENT KINDS OF POST-TRAUMATIC STRESS — SIMPLE AND COMPLEX

It's become clear that *simple post-traumatic stress* resulting from a one-time incident — such as a rape or a serious car accident — is markedly different from the complex set of responses that follows chronic, multiple and/or ongoing traumatic events. Such events include chronic childhood abuse or prolonged experiences of assault and violence in an intimate relationship (for example, violence perpetrated by a spouse or caregiver).

Judith Herman (1992) explains that prolonged repeated trauma occurs in situations where a person is captive, unable to flee, or is under the control of the perpetrator. These conditions render the person powerless and allow the perpetrator *ongoing coercive control*. Such conditions may be found in situations varying from prison camps, some religious cults and conditions of war to some families, or institutions such as residential schools.

Captivity can be achieved by physical force, as with prisoners of war, or by a combination of physical, economic, social and psychological means, as is typically the case for battered women and abused children. The result of this ongoing coercive control is psychological trauma that differs greatly, in complexity and range of effects, from that resulting from a one-time traumatic event. As a result, a new diagnosis has been developed, called *complex PTSD*.

Although this new diagnosis has not yet been officially recognized in the DSM-IV (the fourth and current edition of the *Diagnostic and Statistical Manual of Mental Disorders*, the most-used guide to diagnosing mental health problems), it is currently captured under the general DSM-IV category of "Disorders of Extreme Stress Not Otherwise Specified." This is an important

Recognizing, consciousness-raising around and "naming," the violence in women's lives is an important part of understanding the nature of this experience.

It's not enough, though, to merely identify violence in women's lives. Front-line workers must help women understand that seemingly unrelated mental health problems are actually responses to — and attempts to cope with — the psychological and physiological disruptions caused by abuse-related trauma. Some of the signs of trauma are anxiety, sleeplessness, depression, eating disorders, self-harming behaviour and agitation.

In many cases, women don't recognize the effects of abuse-related trauma in themselves, yet they struggle in their daily lives to cope with their distress in its hidden forms.

As a result, some women believe they are "crazy" because they can't make sense of the effects of trauma in their lives, and can't connect these effects to earlier traumatic events they've experienced.

As front-line, first-contact workers, you can learn to recognize some of the common effects of post-traumatic stress. You can help these women find help and work toward healing from abuse-related trauma.

Women are about twice as likely as men to develop post-traumatic stress. This is probably because women are much more likely to experience interpersonal violence, such as rape, or physical abuse in an intimate relationship, or childhood sexual abuse. Some women have also experienced ongoing and prolonged violence, as is often the case in wife assault or incest. Still other women face ongoing threats of violence and sexual assault as a result of living in a society where violence against women and children is far too widespread.

development in understanding and treating trauma, and complex PTSD is expected to be included in the DSM-V.

Herman (1992) outlines broad areas of psychological disturbance that distinguish complex PTSD from simple PTSD. The first area involves the types of responses or effects, which are more complex, widespread and persistent in complex PTSD (due to the prolonged nature of the trauma). The second area involves the kinds of characteristic personality changes that accompany complex PTSD, including difficulties with relationships and identity. The third area relates to the survivor's increased vulnerability to further victimization, both in the forms of self-harm as well as harm perpetrated by others.

WHY DO WE NEED TO KNOW ABOUT COMPLEX POST-TRAUMATIC STRESS DISORDER?

Many women who seek treatment in mental health clinics have histories of long-term emotional, physical and sexual abuse. Most mental health professionals have previously not understood that prolonged abuse experiences can cause a person to develop a spectrum of complex psychological trauma responses.

Many trauma survivors who sought mental health services have been given more than one diagnosis (at the same time) to describe their difficulties; these include bipolar disorder, schizophrenia-paranoid type and borderline personality disorder. These diagnoses are descriptive labels for symptoms and behaviours, and they emphasize pathology. Traditional psychiatric diagnoses do not consider the context (for example, traumatic events) in which a person may have developed these responses; in other words, many "symptoms" that women exhibit represent their attempts to cope with and adapt to experiences of traumatic stress. These diagnoses focus on what is "wrong" with the person, rather than on what horrible things have happened to the person.

These multiple diagnoses have serious consequences for treatment: therapy and other treatments can rarely be successful when the underlying issues of trauma and neglect are not identified or addressed.

Research conducted on a sample of people diagnosed with complex PTSR found that those who sought treatment typically had histories of prolonged and/or multiple traumatic experiences (van der Kolk, in press).

Simple post-traumatic stress responses include intrusive re-experiencing of the trauma, numbing and *hyperarousal* (excessive physiological arousal such as insomnia, startle reaction, and irritability). The people who had histories of prolonged abuse or multiple traumas experienced not only the effects of simple PTSR, but also had a variety of other psychological problems, characteristic of complex PTSR.

These additional problems included:
- depression and self-hatred
- significant difficulties dealing with emotions and impulses (also known as *affect dysregulation*), including aggression against themselves
- dissociative responses (such as depersonalization)
- self-destructive behaviour (substance use problems, eating disorders)
- inability to develop and maintain satisfying personal relationships
- a loss of meaning and hope.

FEATURES OF COMPLEX PTSD

Changes in affect regulation (the ability to manage feelings and impulses)
- explosive or extremely inhibited anger
- chronic preoccupation with suicide
- self-injury

Changes in consciousness
- *amnesia* (loss of memory) or *hypermnesia* (heightened recall) for traumatic events
- transient episodes of *dissociation* (losing conscious awareness of the "here and now;" a feeling of "spacing out")
- *depersonalization* (the experience of feeling like an outside observer of one's mental processes or body; e.g., feeling like one is in a dream)
- *derealization* (feeling that the external world is altered, unfamiliar or unreal; e.g., people seem unfamiliar or time may seem sped up or slowed down).
- reliving disturbing experiences with intrusive images or thoughts

Changes in self-perception
- sense of helplessness
- shame, guilt and self-blame
- sense of stigma
- sense of difference from others

Changes in perception of perpetrator
- preoccupation with relationship with perpetrator
- attributing total power to perpetrator
- idealizing or, paradoxically, feeling gratitude toward perpetrator
- accepting belief system or rationalization of perpetrator

Changes in relationships
- isolation and withdrawal
- disruption in intimate relationships
- repeated search for rescuer
- persistent distrust

Changes in systems of meaning
- loss of sustaining faith
- loss of hope
- sense of despair

Changes in the body due to psychological and emotional distress (somatization)
- the expression of emotional distress through physical difficulties such as headaches, chronic pain, gastrointestinal problems, etc.

The people interviewed in this study said it was these problems, rather than the effects of simple post-traumatic stress, that created the most psychological distress for them and prompted them to seek help.

Childhood abuse and complex PTSD

The impact of trauma depends on many things. In cases of abuse in childhood, the overall impact depends on developmental issues, such as the age at which the child abuse began; the nature, severity and duration of the abuse; and the relationship of the perpetrator.

The impact also depends on whether the abuse took place in a larger context of severe neglect and *emotional invalidation*. Emotional invalidation means that a person's feelings, such as anger, distress, or hurt, are not attributed to the harmful or abusive events. Instead, for example, the feelings are minimized or the person is accused of being "over-sensitive" or "paranoid."

Chronic abuse in childhood — on its own or combined with a lack of *emotionally connected parenting* (being able to recognize and respond appropriately to a child's emotional state) — profoundly shapes and negatively affects a person's cognitive, emotional, and psychosocial development. These negative effects are worsened when childhood abuse occurs in an environment where a child is also deprived of essential emotional needs, such as safety, constancy and emotional validation.

Adults who grow up with these types of childhoods are most likely to develop complex PTSR. They will likely experience a host of psychological problems, including:
- low self-esteem
- feeling that they are bad or not worthy
- difficulty forming and maintaining relationships
- out-of-control emotional responses

- a tendency to become easily overwhelmed and disorganized by relatively small stressors
- engaging in self-destructive behaviour, such as substance use and other self-harming practices.

Women with a history of childhood physical, sexual or emotional abuse or neglect may develop PTSR when faced with an additional trauma later in life, such as sexual assault, abuse by a partner, divorce or loss of a loved one.

For reasons of clarity, throughout the rest of this guide the discussion will mainly refer to post-traumatic stress responses (PTSR), to capture the various types of post-traumatic stress (simple and complex).

TRAUMA IN A BIOPSYCHOSOCIAL FRAMEWORK

Trauma can change a person's life when it leads to disruptions in emotion, consciousness, memory, sense of self, attachment to others and relationships. What's more, trauma doesn't just affect women's minds. It affects their bodies as well. Responses of the body are known as *physiological* responses. When children are abused by their own caretakers, or while sleeping in their own beds, they cannot fight or flee. They are often trapped physically by the perpetrator, trapped emotionally by their attachment to the perpetrator or else they are made powerless by their mistaken beliefs that they are to blame for the abuse. Similarly, many adult women are trapped in relationships with abusive men — they may fear their abusers will kill them if they attempt to leave.

When a person is trapped, his or her sympathetic nervous system is activated. As a result, they often have a surge of physiological arousal — with no outlet for this arousal — resulting in agitation, tension and anxiety.

Prolonged trauma increases and generalizes physiological arousal. Trauma survivors often complain that they are not able to establish a state of calm or comfort. Instead, they too often feel chronically anxious, agitated and tense. This increased physiological arousal often results in insomnia, tension headaches, gastrointestinal disturbances, and back and pelvic pain.

Traumatic experiences, therefore, alter the functioning of the central nervous system as well as general physiological functioning. In this way, trauma has both emotional and physical effects.

Trauma is best discussed in a framework that takes into account the physiological and psychological levels on which trauma is experienced, as well as the social context in which the trauma occurs. This is known as the *biopsychosocial framework*.

In this biopsychosocial framework, all responses to trauma are understood as attempts to cope with the stress of trauma. People adapt — mentally, physically, behaviourally and socially — to traumatic experiences. The social context and circumstances that define and shape girls' and women's lives also shape the ways they cope with trauma.

Powerlessness in society

When a child's bodily autonomy and integrity and sense of *efficacy* (sense of competence and ability to make things happen) are harmed by experiences of childhood abuse or neglect, the child is rendered powerless *(disempowerment)*.

Feelings of powerlessness are increased when a child is fearful, unable to have adults validate her hurtful experience, and when she realizes that her dependence on adults has her trapped in the abusive situation.

The use of force and threat are not even necessary in many cases of child abuse, especially when the abuse is perpetrated by trusted family members. The fear of losing a life-sustaining relationship is threatening enough for a child.

Most children respond to this experience of disempowerment and entrapment by accommodating the needs of the abuser. They learn to comply with whatever their abuser expects of them, in hopes of avoiding further abuse or rejection. They learn that it is not safe to assert their own needs and will.

Too often, mental health providers do not fully understand the social and psychological factors that shape these adaptations and responses in women's lives. As a result, mental health providers may be impatient with trauma survivors, perceiving them as "chronic victims" who should just learn to assert themselves. This failure to understand can make women feel further blamed, and ashamed for the ways they have tried to protect themselves and manage.

For many women, disempowerment doesn't end when they are free of their childhood abusers. They often have an ongoing experience of disempowerment because of gender inequality, racism, and poverty in their lives. Gender inequality, in which women are seen as having a lesser social value, often causes women to feel powerless, vulnerable and at the mercy of others. This social disempowerment then shapes and intensifies a woman's reaction to being abused.

The social conditions of many women's lives help keep them fearful, *hypervigilant* (always on the lookout for danger), disempowered and vulnerable. As well, inequality affects mental health and can exacerbate the long-term effects of abuse in childhood. For example, women who face ongoing racism, homophobia, sexism or conditions of poverty may respond by using coping strategies such as hypervigilance or *disconnection* (taking themselves mentally out of a situation), because they are triggered by these threatening and disempowering experiences.

Abuse survivors are often told their experiences are in the past, and they should no longer feel the same need for self-protection. However, the reality is that many women are still vulnerable and exposed to ongoing violence and social marginalization, especially lesbians, women of colour, women with disabilities, and women living in poverty.

The responses to these experiences include ongoing depression or sleeping disorders. Many women adapt by disconnecting through self-harm or the use of medication, alcohol and other drugs.

The role of front-line workers

As a critical first step, front-line workers can play an important role in addressing issues of safety in women's lives. Women who have post-traumatic stress cannot reap much benefit from therapeutic interventions when they don't have a safe place to live or enough money to survive.

An important part of understanding trauma, therefore, involves recognizing and understanding the effects of social inequality on women. It also means that *psychoeducational supportive counselling* (education on psychological responses and processes) and help with basic needs are important parts of working with trauma and women with post-traumatic stress.

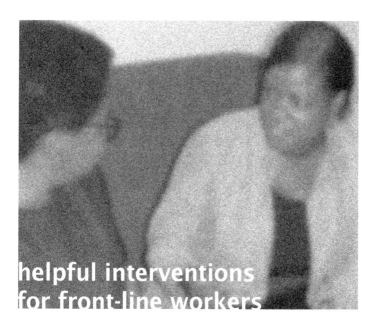

helpful interventions for front-line workers

WHAT CAN YOU OFFER AS A FRONT-LINE WORKER?
For effective intervention and support, it is critical to identify post-traumatic stress in women's lives. Front-line trauma interventions are not restricted to identifying and referring clients to therapy. They also include psychoeducational supportive counselling and help gaining access to basic resources. Appropriate intervention is important in treating PTSR. You can facilitate recovery by integrating the following guidelines into your routine practice:

- Learn to recognize and identify post-traumatic stress reactions.
- Screen for indicators of past trauma or PTSR through routine history-taking.
- Explore the possibility of PTSR as an underlying problem when appropriate.
- Reframe "symptoms" as "adaptations" or "coping strategies" to trauma. This helps to de-stigmatize these responses.
- Understand and explain that reacting to and coping with

trauma is a normal response to an abnormal event. Help women understand that dissociation, emotional numbing and self-harm are their ways of adapting and coping with the overwhelming effects of trauma. It helps normalize the responses.
· Offer support by providing information on post-traumatic stress and the effects of violence.
· Be familiar with local referral options for therapy or support, and direct trauma survivors to referrals when needed. Referrals need to include resources for women's basic needs, such as food, shelter, clothing, physical health and income supports.

RECOGNIZING THE SIGNS OF POST-TRAUMATIC STRESS RESPONSES

Women with PTSR often seek medical care for a range of healthcare problems for which past trauma may be the real underlying or a contributing cause. PTSR is not always recognized, because other problems can mask or intensify PTSR. These problems might include, for example, insomnia, depression, eating disorders, pelvic pain, chronic fatigue and/or fibromyalgia, migraine headaches, irritable bowel syndrome and substance use problems. In many cases, health-care professionals misdiagnose the PTSR because the traumatic cause of the "problems" has not been recognized. To be more effective in the services and support we offer women, we need to adopt the practice of systematic screening for trauma and PTSR as part of the regular history-taking process.

Post-traumatic stress often appears with physiological as well as psychological responses. Some of the most common of these may include:

Mental health problems
- depression
- chronic difficulties sleeping
- *dissociation* (losing conscious awareness of the "here and now"; a feeling of "spacing out")
- *depersonalization* (feeling like an outside observer of one's own body or mental processes)
- *derealization* (the external world seems unfamiliar or unreal)
- anxiety disorders, such as panic attacks

Impaired sense of self
- shame, guilt and self-blame
- self-hate and self-loathing
- damaged, defiled or stigmatized
- helpless or paralyzed in terms of taking initiative
- completely different from others (may include a sense of being special, being utterly alone, or a belief that no other person can understand them)

Relationship difficulties
- unable to trust others
- frequent conflicts
- not feeling entitled to set boundaries
- repeated search for rescuer (may alternate with isolation and withdrawal)
- sexual difficulties
- unable to develop and maintain close attachments
- experiences of revictimization (adult sexual assault, involvement with physically or emotionally abusive partners)
- issues with sexual identity

Problems with memory
- gaps in memories of childhood
- difficulty remembering discussions from the previous week
- amnesia or intense recollection of traumatic events

Behavioural expressions of distress
- problems with alcohol or drug use
- suicidal impulses
- self-inflicted harm
- eating disorders
- shoplifting
- high-risk sexual behaviours that may result in unintended pregnancy or sexually transmitted diseases

Physical problems
- chronic pain with no medical basis (often gynecological problems in women)
- stress-related conditions, such as chronic fatigue syndrome or fibromyalgia
- headaches
- sleep disorders
- breathing problems or asthma

HOW TO SCREEN FOR POST-TRAUMATIC STRESS RESPONSES

The following are suggestions on how to ask about possible traumatic experiences and responses when conducting a history-gathering interview. The focus of the questions can be modified, depending on the situation.

To establish a rapport and offer comfort to clients, keep in mind a few basic principles.

Practice active facilitation.
When a front-line worker, or anyone in a helping role, sits with a survivor and hears her despair and pain, and remains silent, many survivors will feel even more fear and shame.

In listening to a survivor describe her experiences, active facilitation is the appropriate response. Active facilitation is the process of offering active and respectful engagement, and providing sensitive and nuanced responses to what is being said.

WHEN ASKING CLIENTS ABOUT THEIR EXPERIENCES,

- React so clients understand how you are thinking and feeling about what they are disclosing. Make a direct statement, such as: "I now understand why you feel [specify feeling]." Or say: "What a horrible experience to have lived through." This kind of statement reflects your empathic reactions, whereas simply asking the client, "How did this experience make you feel?" asks her to disclose more information to you without receiving any reassuring feedback.
- Be familiar with *reframing statements* and *normalizing* comments. For example, if a woman tells you she never tells anyone about her past experiences of abuse, you could say: "That is a way you try to keep yourself protected from being hurt by the other people's lack of knowledge about these difficult experiences."
- Highlight interpersonal strengths and supports. For example, help a woman see her accomplishments in the face of the abuse: "You were able to *not* accept [the perpetrator's] definition of you [use the client's own example; e.g., that you were "useless"] and in fact you provided good care and support to your children."

Normalize the process.
Incorporate questions about past or present trauma as a part of all personal history assessments. Make it clear that all clients are asked these questions routinely. Ask questions about possible traumatic experiences in a relaxed and matter-of-fact manner. This will decrease the likelihood that the client will feel singled out and stigmatized.

Reframe negative symptoms.
Describe them instead as understandable adaptations, coping strategies and self-protective behaviours.

ACTIVELY FACILITATING ABUSE DISCLOSURES: FINDING THE BALANCE

Active facilitation enables you to be present and self-aware in the interview, and to be engaged and empathic without being intrusive. Clients experience questions as intrusive if they are asked in a demanding way or with a tone of judgment or disbelief.

Asking someone about her experiences of abuse or neglect is a finely balanced process. The front-line worker asks questions in a relaxed manner — not in a hushed or indifferent tone. It's also important to get permission to ask more questions (e.g., "Is it okay if we talk about this a bit more?").

Some people avoid asking questions about abuse because they believe it's a violation of the client's privacy. They may also be afraid of causing the client emotional pain or discomfort. This approach, however, leaves trauma survivors alone, isolated and silenced. Most people are relieved when asked about their experiences in a relaxed and straightforward way.

It's critically important, however, that you don't make the following mistakes when asking about trauma and abuse:
- When validating the client's experience of violation, don't make sweeping statements about abuse. For example, many clients blame themselves, and believe they actively participated or were complicit in the abuse. As a result, they may interpret statements, such as "abuse is wrong," to mean they have done something bad. Offer more nuanced responses to explain the harm of abuse, such as:

    "What was done to you was wrong."
    "Children can never consent to sex with an adult."
    "Children often accommodate unwanted sexual acts as a way to survive what was done to them."

- Don't burden the client with your own revelations or with your own strong or extreme responses. Again, the balance is important to find. At times, it's appropriate and helpful to tell the trauma survivor that you've talked with many women who have similar experiences of abuse, but don't share examples of other women's experiences. It's also inappropriate to express anger at the person who perpetrated the abuse. Many survivors haven't comes to terms with their own anger, and may feel alienated by your response or feel a need to protect the perpetrator.

Remember: this may be the first time anyone has asked the client about these experiences. A positive and respectful experience may encourage clients to consider further professional help. It's important to ask these questions, but be respectful if the woman isn't able to discuss these issues. Let her know you are open to talking about this again in the future.

HELPFUL QUESTIONS FOR POST-TRAUMATIC STRESS RESPONSE SCREENING

Here are some questions about past or present trauma that you can ask clients. These are suggestions and can be modified to suit your service or personal style.

Introduce questions with a statement.
"I ask the following questions of all of the people I work with, because the things we experience in life can very often have an impact on our health."

Ask respectful questions.
"How are things going with your family?"
"How is your relationship going?"
"Have you ever had a traumatic experience in your life? For example, have you ever been hurt or injured? Have you ever felt that your life was in danger?"
"Have you ever been mistreated or harmed by someone you care about?" (like a family member or a partner)
"Has anything very upsetting happened to you recently? What about the more distant past?"
"Did you find it difficult to cope with this experience?"
"Are there things in your life now that worry you?"
"Have you ever been forced into a sexual experience that you didn't want?"

Give your sense of the situation based on the answers to these questions. Also include your observations about any responses they may be experiencing.
"I've noticed that [specify your observation], and I wonder if this is what's going on?"

"I'm not sure about your situation, but from what you've said to me, it may be that some of the ways in which you cope may have been learned from an experience in your past that was traumatic."

Ask questions that may help determine the presence of PTSR.
"Are there things from your past that still bother you in an ongoing way?"
"Do you sometimes have the same upsetting dreams?"
"Are there details about your past that you find difficult to remember?"
"Do you feel connected and close to your family and friends?" Or: "Do you feel isolated?"
"Do you still take pleasure in the activities you've always enjoyed?"
"Do you have trouble sleeping? Either getting to sleep, or sleeping through the night?"
"Do you feel on edge?"
"Do you feel upset in your everyday life (for example, at work or in your family)?"

BE PREPARED FOR AND BE SENSITIVE TO CLIENTS' RESPONSES

Remember that a client may become upset or agitated talking about these painful issues.

If a client becomes upset discussing these issues, it doesn't mean you have traumatized her. Many people avoid asking about trauma and abuse. They think it's too upsetting for clients. In reality, it's often the person in the helping role who is uncomfortable or inexperienced in dealing with normal reactions to talking about trauma.

It's important to acknowledge that you are sorry she is upset, but don't apologize for asking the questions. These questions are important — suggesting it's wrong to ask them undermines your effort. The client may also think your apology means it's bad or shameful to discuss trauma and abuse.

Offer a referral for professional help or services, and/or a follow-up appointment after you discuss such issues with the client.

It's important to explain to clients that relief is possible and that there are many available therapies.

> **NOTE**
>
> *Avoid asking these screening questions unless you are prepared to offer referrals for appropriate services.*
>
> *Do not probe women's trauma memories or explore them any further than is required to screen for a history of trauma. Many survivors of severe childhood abuse require an initial and often lengthy period of therapy to develop fundamental skills before they begin exploring their childhood trauma.*
>
> However, in the event that a woman discloses details of her abuse experience, don't cut her off. This may shame and silence her, and she may not discuss her experiences in the future. Listen and respond with validating statements. Acknowledge what a painful experience it must have been. Give her a referral to a professionally trained therapist who can provide ongoing therapy. If that makes her uncomfortable, tell her she can meet with you again; however, explain that you are unable to offer therapy but can provide support and assistance.

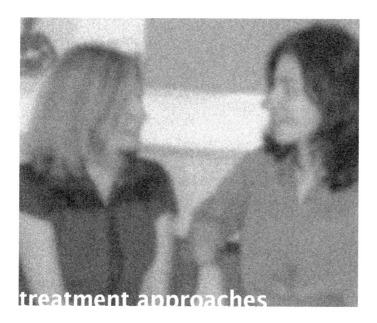

treatment approaches

THERAPEUTIC OPTIONS

Fortunately, there are a variety of treatments for PTSR. Treatment usually involves some form of psychotherapy, and may also include medication, at least for a period of time.

Research has demonstrated that there are specific psychotherapy approaches and techniques that are especially effective in treating PTSR. For this reason, it's important to find qualified and professionally trained therapists who are experienced in providing specialized trauma therapy.

Generally, psychotherapy or psychoanalysis that probes and explores trauma memories is not considered helpful and may in fact be harmful. These forms of psychotherapy may cause clients to become overwhelmed with traumatic responses, memories and feelings before they are able to tolerate them.

Therapeutic approaches that are considered the most effective include: cognitive behaviour therapy (including exposure and anxiety techniques); eye movement, desensitization and reprocessing therapy (known as EMDR); some body therapies; and some psychoeducational group therapies specifically geared to dealing with trauma.

Therapy for trauma survivors should be phase-oriented. The initial stage should focus on helping survivors manage responses and increase their safety, and on psychoeducation about trauma and its after-effects. For more information on therapy for trauma survivors, see Lori Haskell's *First Stage Trauma Treatment: A Guide for Therapists Working with Women* (in press), also published by the Centre for Addiction and Mental Health (listed in the references at the back of this guide).

WHEN MEDICATION MIGHT BE HELPFUL

When people have been identified as having PTSR, they can, in many cases, experience relief from the responses with the aid of medication. These responses, which can be overwhelming, include sleeplessness, depression and panic attacks. It's important to refer clients to psychiatrists and medical doctors who have specific expertise in the appropriate treatments for complex PTSR.

THE IMPORTANCE OF REFERRALS

Once front-line workers start screening for trauma in the lives of women at your service, you will likely be astounded with the frequency of the disclosures and the need to find suitable therapy.

Develop a list of qualified organizations and resources to which you can refer clients. It may help to contact the organizations and ask about their services, whether they have waiting lists, whether they offer individual or group therapy and what stage of trauma treatment they offer.

COLLABORATIVE APPROACHES

Some services for women may want to team up with a trained trauma therapist. Rather than refer women individually for therapy (which is not always available or affordable), the service can have the trauma therapist conduct skill-based therapy groups that provide women with basic tools they need to cope with trauma, such as being able to:
- separate the past from the present (grounding)
- exercise control and choice
- stay connected or regain connection to positive others
- recognize, whenever possible, the connection between past experiences and present behaviours and feelings.

For example, some addiction services recognize that many women who have substance use problems also have a history of trauma and abuse. These services collaborate with specially trained trauma therapists to provide on-site specialized groups for women dealing with these complex issues.

A HOPEFUL CONCLUDING NOTE

Fortunately, a great deal has been learned about post-traumatic stress in the last several years. There are increasingly effective ways to offer support and relief. As a result, many people can be helped with the appropriate treatment, especially if there is early recognition and intervention.

In working with women who are coping with trauma, it's important to offer hope. As service providers who often have first contact with women experiencing post-traumatic stress, you play a critical role in identifying the signs. You can also offer support to clients who experience post-traumatic stress, and facilitate referrals for specialized therapeutic help for healing and recovery.

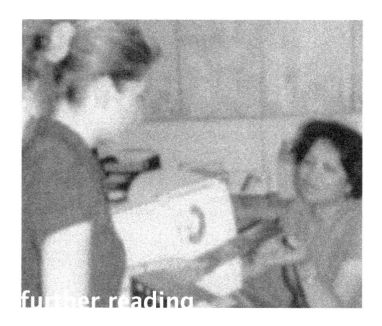

FOR UNDERSTANDING TRAUMA

Allen, J. (1995). *Coping with Trauma: A Guide to Self-Understanding.* Washington, DC: American Psychiatric Press. This is a comprehensive book, written in plain English, that covers some essential topics, including the nature of trauma, its range of biological, psychological and relational effects, and treatment.

Haskell, L. (in press). *First Stage Trauma Treatment: A Guide for Therapists Working with Women.* Toronto: Centre for Addiction and Mental Health.

Herman, J. (1992). *Trauma and Recovery.* New York: Basic Books.
This is the classic text in which Herman first introduced the concept of complex PTSD, outlined the nature of trauma and explained the process of healing from it.

SOURCES FOR SURVIVORS
Napier, N. (1993). *Getting Through the Day.* New York: W.W. Norton.
This is an especially useful resource for understanding and managing dissociative adaptations.

REFERENCES
American Psychiatric Association. (1994). *Diagnostic and Statistical Manual of Mental Disorders* (4th ed.). Washington, DC: Author.

Herman, J. (1992). *Trauma and Recovery.* New York: Basic Books.

van der Kolk, B.A. (in press). The assessment and treatment of complex PTSD. In R. Yehuda (Ed.), *Traumatic Stress* (Chapter 7). Washington, DC: American Psychiatric Press.

Lightning Source UK Ltd.
Milton Keynes UK
UKHW050524090920
369560UK00009B/190